Transition
Thunderstorms

Beth Bonness

A Publication of The Poetry Box®

Editing & Book Design by Shawn Aveningo Sanders
Cover Design by Shawn Aveningo Sanders
  (using photograph of tree by Beth Bonness)
Author Photo by Sarah Eastlund

ISBN: 978-1-956285-07-9
Printed in the United States of America.
Wholesale distribution via Ingram.

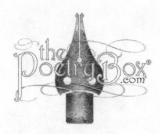

Published by The Poetry Box®, April 2022
Portland, Oregon
https://ThePoetryBox.com

*To my husband, Jeff, and our three daughters:
Kalah, Rachel, and Amanda — they kept me anchored
while navigating my thunderstorms.*

Contents

wrong word dinner

robe of white wraps around my recovering body
my husband and daughters' dinner table chatter surrounds me
leftovers warm in the microwave
everyone's smiling

today's been a better day
blood pressure's holding
read a bit of a book
sleep's been okay

longer concentration than yesterday
journaled with less frustration…yet
my 'o's and 'e's and 'a's still collapse
deflated helium balloons in my cursive

the girls chatter on about their day
peppered with questions from dad
my private ping-pong game
keep up with their conversations

lean in for a question—
my lips part…
    by the time a thought is firm
    the girls are off to their next topic
…my lips close
forced smile intact

no reason to let them know
i'm having trouble keeping up
though they sense it…
when they ask me a question
their pace slows

B*E*E*P

husband's chair scrapes and squeals on the floor
as he starts to rise i pop up before he does
wrapping my white robe sash tighter
the microwave door swings open

words in my head stand in line ready for their turn
only they get all mixed up when they come out
like someone at camp stopping abruptly
an entire line of words falling over each other

middle daughter points to an apple
i say *orange*
the word apple mute at the back of my brain
in the shadows
her buddy orange answers on apple's behalf

youngest daughter points to her water glass
i say *chair*
my smile collapses
joined by their smiles weakening

…not again…
no evil snowflakes in my peripheral vision
this time
no hand claw
…only wrong words…

hunger disappears
adrenaline fills my belly
tears well up
don't want the girls
to see me like this
—*stop talking*
      then you won't say the wrong word

slip away into the living room
lights off
laughter from moments earlier
disintegrates into murmurs

too much excitement
stay still for a bit
doctor's orders
—meds and rest—
the house is quiet
—meds and rest—
tears fall onto my white robe
invisible
i don't stop them
until i hear footsteps

my youngest crouches down
her hands on my knees
voice gentle

...mama
you know you have to go back to the hospital
don't you...

her 15 year eyes
searching for recognition
in my almost 50 year ones

when did our roles reverse?
i shake my head yes

upstairs to change
with all my wrong words
mashing around in my head
unable to get out
in the order right

these hands

my wrinkly hands...mostly from age
partly from bad choices with the sun
these hands have typed on typewriters, computer keyboards,
    and teletype machines
(what are those things again? wait...how old am i?)
these hands have changed diapers and made bread
caressed my husband's curly hair when it was black and our
    daughters' red cheeks
chopped 1000s of carrots and potatoes, sliced skin off fingertips,
    held babies
checked and signed homework, driven cars
held movie tickets and main sheets, held water ski ropes and
    climbing lines
typed and retyped hateful responses, deleted the digital echoes
washed out swimming suits and torn junk mail for handmade
    paper
cut mensural blood stains from the lining of a long winter coat
brushed the girls' hair, painted their fingernails
held up drywall sheets and painted walls
'borrowed' money from my mother's wallet to buy presents as a
    kid
rubbed sleepies from the girls' eyes and rubbed suntan lotion on
    their backs
raked leaves, moved laws, and weeded
prepared Chinese, Indian, and Italian food, slushes and
    cappuccinos
flapped and lain still
dismissed someone sharing their story, burned knuckles
    simmering some stock
done wash, ironed sheets, and first communion dresses
clapped and wiped away tears
retaken post-stroke high blood pressure until numbers came
    down, hid stats from my docs
held babies when getting vaccines, sprayed water on them when
    too hot

watered plants and washed floors
dropped wine glasses after drinking too much
changed oil and conked out using stick shift on a hill
forgot turn signals and pissed people off
held harnesses during skydiving and folded tents on vacation
tested bathwater and baby bottles
taken temperatures and changed tires
gone grocery shopping, held tight on roller coaster rides, tied
    little shoes
clipped nails and played cards
not picked up my cellphone while driving home late
done puzzles and practiced piano
swatted mosquitoes and let spiders loose
brushed webs aside and pushed sunglasses up
flossed teeth and organized vitamins
written checks and paid street musicians
lit candles in quiet meditation and on romantic getaways
cut umbilical cords and held mother-in-law's dying hands
these hands, my hands
they hold my memories

thanksgiving
with a side of no thank-you #1

my arm won't move
i can't feel my
left arm!
no, I feel it
i feel tingles
like the one
you have when
your arm falls asleep
then wakes up with little
nibbling minnows screaming
their sharp teeth under your skin
although the screaming is
silent, but you can feel it
swell from inside
your arm

is my left hand a claw?

or only stiff from circulation
being cut off to my arm because
i slept on it too long
there aren't any evil
snowflakes in my
peripheral
vision

i wish the damn beeping telemetry machine
would SHUT UP—take a break
i'd still be here when you got back

back dive

my arms ex...tend strAight over head
elbows locked at attention
thumbs cross-crossed in a butterfly bridge
fingers glued together, point to the sky
ten feet above the water
teeth chatter
locks of hair escape the
t.i.g.h.t
white
latex
bathing caP
smothering my ears,
what is my instructor saying?
arch backwards
my heart races
legs s•h.a•••K,e
chlorinated crystals
d
...r
......
......i
.........p
from the little red riBBons
on my *ladylike* navy bLue
polYESter
one-piece
bathing suit
with a white p•L.e•A.t•E.d skirt
hyper-XtENDed toes
g•r•i•pp•ING
a sun-bleached powder-blue board
scratT.chy
non-stICK gooseBUMP sandpaper
heels overlooking the calm water below
look up at your fingertips

[. . .]

eyes glued to my instrUctor's eyes
a foot away
three inches shorter
his hands behind my back
it's oKay
holding me steady
I won't let go until you're ready
the sun burns as i peek uP
i'm hOlding my breath
eyes clOsed
nod
arm brace reLEASed

F•••
A•••
L•••
L•••
I•••
N•••
G

b
a
c
k
w
a
r
d
s

...SPLA••shh
disappearing
into the c.Old water
muffled voices above
SINk
•••••ing
holding my breath
eyes O.P.en
feet touch the rough bottom
crouched down
arms overhead
heels and toes thrust uP...WARD
arms cooperate in reaching for air
EX.hale
smile broaD•L•••Y

thanksgiving
with a side of no thank-you #2

i'm wearing one of those washed too many times
paper-thin, ugly greenish-blue hospital gowns
with preschool geometric patterns
you find on airport carpets
created by somebody
who flunked
design
school
predictable
and boring as
muzak in elevators
that makes you want
to take the stairs versus listen
so you try to blot out the sound
with your thoughts relegating it to
white noise, you'd prefer to be silent
why aren't i wearing my pajamas in the hospital?

you don't wear pajamas

i would prefer one of jeff's shirts
anything
but this wrapping paper screaming

SICK PERSON
SICK PERSON

the night she died

i peer through the upstairs railing
our front door open, mom stands
in her white puffy robe in the
middle of the night, dad is next
to her, his back to me, he holds
my little sister's body, her three-
year-old head nestled in his left
elbow, a lace bonnet with blond
curls scotch-taped inside
her legs to his right...still...

in the driveway
a police car idles, lights off
an officer escorts my father
clutching her tiny frame toward
the car, dad slips in the backseat
cradling my sister, adjusting her
bonnet, the squad door closes
we watch them drive away, mom
and i, she closes the front door
cutting off cold air, replacing the
warmth of my littlest sister

thanksgiving
with a side of no thank-you #3

in a private room this time
what time is it?
6:30, 7 AM?
where's the
nurse?
damn,
there
goes
the
blood
pressure
machine
waking
up
again

*pum**hiss**P*
*pum**hiss**P*

the velcro sleeve
slapped around
my bicep
as i tried
to sleep
all night
crunches
my
pressure
builds…stretching
the sticky & soft parts
trying to separate them

stop holding your breath
it only makes the numbers go up

                              i can't
                    my heart's racing too fast

breathe deeply
...in...
...out...

                    my arm still tingles

wedding thunderstorms

smiling at me from
high above an oregon beach
clouds waft past, dripping
their mist onto the waves

rainbow-bubble reflections
float on the wind
past the windows
while drinking champagne
and eating m&ms
lined up by color

my personal guilty pleasure
where did all the brown ones go?
there used to be more
now blue, my favorite color
seems to be the queen

popping them in two at a time
one for each cheek
sucking them until the
chocolate shell melts
can't wait that long
crunch and chew

the chocolate of my childhood
along with toll house cookies
216 for my husband
then boyfriend's 18th birthday

1500 for our wedding
overlooking madison's lake mendota
wearing a one-size fits all
wedding dress
my husband, then fiancee
found on the cover of a cosmopolitan magazine
while waiting in line at the grocery store
months before we wed

on the day, a private moment
before hundreds of guests
under a beautiful blue sky
after morning thunderstorm clouds
threatened to roll in again
i swam in the aquamarine lake
reflecting the sky

bewildering the women
watching from their hotel rooms
beneath a sky riddled with
thunderclouds, as it should be
for a wedding

thanksgiving
with a side of no thank-you #4

i spot people outside my door
through the little window
coffee mixed with
antiseptic soap
passes

a new nurse
shoulders the door open
"you're awake, good morning"

left arm doesn't work!
left arm doesn't work!

she can't hear me
tears well up in my eyes

don't cry
don't cry

"you okay honey?"
i shrug my shoulders
she checks the bp reading
"let's try again"

must be high

"you okay?"
i shake my head no
"want me to call somebody?"

YES, i want you to call jeff
but he finally got a good night's sleep
i don't want to wake him up

or scare him

she can't hear me
i shake my head yes
she slips out the door
faster than she eased in
once the door closes tears fall
sunrise crimson and coral peep through
the partially open window slats
swaying when the heat is on
it was daylight most of the
night inside my room
with the backlit
mood lighting
behind my
bed
out of reach
to turn off, only
it wouldn't because
like generator lighting
it's always on, wouldn't want
any of the doctors (or nurses) to
trip when they didn't tiptoe into my
room to check on me during the night

be nice
they're trying to figure out what's happening to you
okay

9 o'clock

```
                overhead
          roam         tum
        storms              bling
       der                  away
     thun                   before
     m[in                        cir
       side]e              cling
       started             back
            they      to
           where
```

thanksgiving
with a side of no thank-you #5

today's thanksgiving
our new french friends
were going to celebrate
with our old portland friends
our three daughters home from
school and work for a long weekend
only we left all the food in a couple of
safeway grocery carts when i started
seeing evil snowflakes yesterday
out of the corner of my left eye
like the night i had my first
tia, my first transitory
ischemic attack

my first 'warning stroke'
after you have a warning stroke the
others can't be called warning strokes

you've been warned

i've been warned

how many have you had so far?

i don't remember
think it's around four

does it matter?

happy 50^b birthday
and you wanted machu picchu

partner

m•e in
w..e

hands hold
together
t.ouch()

walkin.g
talking
liquid silence

decades of pictures
lai.•d
down

spread—. out
slept in—
~- on

washed with coffee
and
wine

spoon•in,g((
roll over
))
enveloped
in —mem,•ory

w..e
sle•e•p

thanksgiving
with a side of no thank-you #6

now i wish the doctors
would figure out
what's causing
the attacks
first, silent
white sparkles
off to my left side
painless pressure pulses
behind my eyeballs
then the words

or lack of words

my inside voice

works fine

but when the main
gatekeeper lets words
out she must be new and
didn't go through enough
training because she lets
whomever rushes to the
front of the line
get out
first
regardless of
my attempting to control
word toddlers jockeying for
position & falling over each
other as they tumble out

[. . .]

better
keep
unpre-
dictble
words
inside
other-
wise
people
might
think

CRAZY PERSON
CRAZY PERSON!

nose piercing

fingers shake ever so slightly
beneath a cupped hand
resting on my lap
smile thoughts forced over a cliff
by inside cheering hooligans
ready for initiation
of a lifetime under
....cover
member
expOsed
it's time...
inked Brooklyn expat
disarming chatter
a purposeful distraction
welcomed
point by point prelude
......
deEP neRvoUs in....HALE
....
...EX...ha...le
quick
cRunCH
through cartilage
tears stre
.............a
...............m
a delayed
JOLT
of adrenaline
arm-crossed hooligans
watching
high-five each other
nostril tWitches
a tiny
diamond
sparkleS

thanksgiving
with a side of no thank-you #7

"your husband is on his way"
guided into an empty wheelchair
"doctor ordered another mri"

my fake
i'm-okay-not-really-but-i'll-pretend smile
implodes

my teeth chatter
my body shakes
uncontrollably
in a tsunami
wave all the
way down
to my
toes

what's happening to me?

clench my left hand
over and over
then my
right
as if
they
were
twins
maybe
my right
can cajole
my left to unfreeze

i want jeff here
now

his strong, calm hazel eyes
to tell me everything is
going to be okay
even though
he never says that
he tells me he loves me
listens even if he can't hear me
he sees something in my eyes
and with words that escape
knows how to fill in the blanks
based on my pantomime

i'll take that please
his familiar face

didn't recognize old-shifters last night
or any new-shifters this morning
tired of being stuck
in the hospital
in a hospital bed
in a hospital gown
with eerie lights
you can never tell
what time it is
'cause the room
looks the same
24 hours a day

i want away from the
constant beeping telemetry
the house-arrest bp cuff

i want the fuck out

[. . .]

don't know what's wrong
if we can't find out what's wrong
we can't stop it

i want it to stop

STOP IT!

whatever IT is

sneezes

ah
choo
goose bumps
pop to
attention
eyes close tight
mid-thought
slight internal
dribble
out my nose
gesundheit
good health
no more god bless you
bless you is
okay, but I prefer
gesundheit
a nod to my german heritage
even though i disown the whole
nazi thing, i prefer to remember
schaum
tortes

thanksgiving
with a side of no thank-you #8

the hospital is sparse because it's a holiday
corridors & elevators dimmed & empty
once down in the basement with the
mri machine a lanky orderly says
"wait here, they beeped someone
on call, shouldn't take too long"
magnetic resonance imaging
people have the day off
except i'm the reason
someone has to come
back, the orderly turns
on the lights in the long
hallway & waiting room even
though i'm the only person there
then lanky scurries back down the hall

no more beeping telemetry machines

silence

except for the elevator bell
announcing this floor and the
THWUMP of the doors closing
try to follow the sound of the car
going up until...i can't hear it anymore
extra silence with a side of heart racing

where's jeff?
how will he know
i'm down here?

after the MRI you can see him

stare at the waiting room usually filled with
family members and worried faces
it's a ghost town this morning
minutes later when i hear
tennis shoes slapping
on speckled linoleum
i spy a woman
in jeans & a t-shirt
hiking toward
me backlit with
an emergency light
she smiles at me
"sorry it took so long
had to drive in
from clackamas,
more symptoms?"

my head sways
waiting for my stumbling words
to accompany my left hand motion
only tingles escape the overbearing gatekeeper
while i massage my left forearm

once inside the mri machine-cave
with a perfect arc inches above my face
the t-shirt woman's voice squawks
through speakers overhead
"try to stay still,
i'd like to get back
for turkey dinner"
with a laugh
no polite laughing from me
she couldn't see my face
only my brain

[. . .]

breathe
breathe

the couldn't-talk-without-screaming
above the loud drum-hum made me want to
curl up under a blanket, my teeth chattered

did that count as moving?
i don't want to be here for turkey dinner either

after thirty minutes
the high-pitched drum-hum starts to slow
like a ferris wheel announcing the ride was over
you're in the last cage
waiting patiently

for

every

one

else

to

be

let

off

first

the t-shirt woman returns & pushes a button
to glide the shelf i shivered on out
she grabbed some thin blankets
placed them on my knees
"good luck"

back in my wheelchair
i watch her skip down the empty hall
her rubber soles squeaking on the clean floor
until i can't hear them anymore

alone
again
in the silence

my arm not as tingly anymore
maybe just slept wrong
cut off my circulation

where's jeff?
i want my turkey dinner too —
take-out from huber's
in my hospital room
in one of jeff's shirts
with the girls

i want jeff
and the girls
without tingles
without beeping
with normal lights
without a side of IT

blood onion

holding the tendril root end of a peeled white onion
my sharp silver blade pierces the outer skin
slice horizontal
peeking sideways
hesitate
not all the way
withdraw under tension
now vertical cuts

rock back and forth, dice into small pieces
on the stressed maple cutting board
a coat of liquid seeps from my eyeballs
magnifies the translucent gems
reflections of light on the weeping juices
eyelids close
drawing the moisture into puddles
in the corners
by the bridge of my nose

sniff
the salty tears are coaxed back inside
a tiny crimson droplet meanders down a stream of juice
spreading like veins
i paused the blade
but not before i pierced my fingertip
sharp spicy intruders rush inside the wound
before i can suck them out

behind the mirror of someone else

black slips out of a car and walks into the living room with a
lit cigar in his mouth, eyeballs blinking in opposite rhythms to
each other, a tray of bacon-covered dates dare you to eat them
as they hover over invisible hands, one Swedish meatball rolls
in leaving slimy slug trails on your fresh white carpet singing an
Italian opera muffled every 20 seconds when her mouth is on the
floor and the neighbors downstairs hear her voice through the
joists like a foghorn in the bay with flashing red traffic lights off-
circuit waving their gigantic arms frantically to protect everyone
from crashing into anyone else or to keep the aliens from
landing their tinfoil hats extending to the moon while a satellite
gets caught on a golden thread-chain of musical notes played a
century before drinking tea from mugs of silence tired from a
night of dream-tours for little children smarter than their parents
but not allowed to speak to strangers, yet with the windows
open their minds escape into the vast openness of possibilities
without worry of babysitters or leftovers or bullies at school or
brushing their teeth, only painting the stars into giant puzzle
pieces and welcoming the bears to come visit and listen to them
dance on the hearts of their grandparents from three generations
ago never imagining a future where their kids' kids would savor
the same sweet chocolate of life slipping past a mountain goat
noshing on pumpkin seeds from a vending machine of goodness
broken by some teenage hooligans tagging too aggressively

because they were showing off for Santa Claus or was it the Tooth Fairy half-naked with desire for the Easter Bunny who was buck-naked next to the angel kissing the devil while singing 'oh my, what a beautiful day it is' as he winked at the spider crawling on the snowman into his Oreo eye socket spinning his magic sticky web of gunk to place underneath the ogre's toenails before the first communion ritual every springtime in Ireland, where did the time go and how long can you keep up with my prodding and pulling with honey in the jet streams of humming or eating tomatoes in Paris with wine dripping from your mouth wiped off by a pirate of Moroccan descent on his way to a boat with a sword, fighting unimagined monsters in the night of tranquility floating on the pond of serenity covering up the dark-side of the moon to somewhere deep inside your soul far away from anyone else getting to know you, peeking out from behind the mirror of someone else while they examined their body and life and history, they knock on the door and discover you watching as they charge after you and you melt into butter on the floor seeping into the woodwork onto a tiny ant on a trail with a hundred others not looking up or sideways only in front of themselves —*quiet don't speak*— but scanning the room for the giant fans out to hear your heartbeat, it's louder than the others different than the others redder than the others where in the hole to the next stop what creature will you morph into next? ask the genie the wizard the shapeshifter for advice as you pass by silently discussing your dilemma of existence and hunger *where is my chocolate and tea and champagne?* you left them back in Paris with your husband who is asleep at the cafe waiting for you to return from the ladies room in Italy, it was quite a leap through the Louis IV door to oblivion dressed in gelato with a wink and a tiny plastic orange translucent little shovel dropping caramel floating to your lips and once in your mouth it descends back to Paris in a kiss to your husband on his red wine lips with a startle of wakedness and then he falls asleep in your arms as you both drift off to a place you pulled out of a hat at a flea market late at night with minstrels singing softly in the background along the Seine.

hooligans

pushing words over a bridge
"that one…it'll get her in trouble"

can't eat and talk at the same time or i cough

jeff laughs
says i'd starve

storm's a coming

Acknowledgments

"nose piercing" first appeared *The Timberline Review*, edited by Peter R. Field & Pam Wells, 55. Portland: Willamette Writers, Inc., 2015.

"behind the mirror of someone else" first appeared in *Fridays on the Boulevard*, edited by Sarah Bokich, 7. Portland: The Attic Institute, 2021.

Special thanks to Shawn Aveningo Sanders at The Poetry Box for help in guiding me through publication of my first chapbook and to Roxanne Colyer for years of her indefatigable patience and support.

Praise for
Transition Thunderstorms

You want to say "apple" and it comes out "orange." Your hand has turned into a useless claw. You hope it has simply fallen asleep, but you suspect you are having a stroke. In *Transition Thunderstorms*, poet Beth Bonness takes us inside the stroke victim's mind with poems playfully organized on the page to show how in the midst of a thunderstorm or a stroke, the normal rules do not apply. Her "thanksgiving with a side of no thank you" poems show the fear and frustration, the outer and inner struggles with rare honesty and clarity. These are spiced with side dishes about sneezes, nose piercing, love, and death to create a delicious feast for the reader.

—Sue Fagalde Lick, president, Oregon Poetry Association, author of *Gravel Road Ahead* and *The Widow at the Piano*

Beth Bonness writes from the depths of her soul's experience. With the finesse of a true poet, she invites the seeker to the pinch point of their pain, then, having walked the path herself, coaxes the reader through to greater understanding and self-acceptance. With extraordinary alchemy, and a shared sense of empathy and relief, Bonness leaves the reader transformed.

Transition Thunderstorms offers breathtaking insights into life events we find hard to talk about with the people we love most. The book is a tender and honest lifeline to reconnection. Her poetry articulates truths of recovery with gentleness and compassion and resonates hope.

—Roxanne Colyer, award-winning artist, writer, and bio-energy healer.

[. . .]

Anyone who has had a stunning body-breakdown can relate to Beth Bonness' exquisitely written journey into (and thru) the thunderstorms in her brain. Her words resonate with fierce beauty, angst and resilience.

—Anne Mendel, award-winning author
of *Etiquette for an Apocalypse*

About the Author

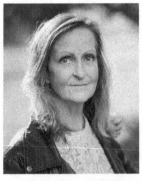

Beth Bonness grew up in Milwaukee, Wisconsin, the eldest of six girls. She moved to the Pacific Northwest with her Computer Science degree and her husband, where they raised their three daughters. She fell in love with the beach and enjoyed climbing Mt. Hood, once. After decades working in product development and marketing (and one too many acquisitions) she said "good-bye" to high-tech corporate culture…to write.

Her poems have appeared in *The Timberline Review*, *Typehouse Magazine*, and *Fridays on the Boulevard*. Two of her short film scripts made it to the Willamette Writers FiLMLaB quarterfinals. She is currently working on a post-stroke memoir about saving a 100-year-old mansion with her husband, and a psychological thriller screenplay about sub-conscious personalities. She lives in Portland, Oregon with her husband and writes early in the morning before she wakes up too much.

LinkedIn: Beth Bonness

Twitter: @BethBonness

Website: bethbonness.com

About The Poetry Box®

The Poetry Box, a boutique publishing company in Portland, Oregon, provides a platform for both established and emerging poets to share their words with the world through beautiful printed books and chapbooks.

Feel free to visit the online bookstore (thePoetryBox.com), where you'll find more titles including:

Exchanging Wisdom by Christopher & Angelo Luna

Sophia & Mister Walter Whitman by Penelope Scambly Schott

Dear John— by Laura LeHew

A Shape of Sky by Cathy Cain

A Long, Wide Stretch of Calm by Melanie Green

Of the Forest by Linda Ferguson

What She Was Wearing by Shawn Aveningo Sanders

The Catalog of Small Contentments by Carolyn Martin

Tell Her Yes by Ann Farley

Sitting in Powell's Watching Burnside Dissolve in the Rain
by Doug Stone

Beneath the Gravel Weight of Stars by Mimi German

A Nest in the Heart by Vivienne Popperl

and more . . .